Health and Fitness Made Easy for Truck Drivers

How to Get in Shape and Live A Healthy Life as A Truck Driver

Nicholas M. Slahta

Introduction

Are you a truck driver, and you feel your weight is getting out of hand?

Have you tried working out, but it feels like you do not have the time to do so owing to your busy schedule?

Is eating healthy while on the road quite challenging?

If the above scenarios describe you, it is time to do something about your situation.

When you are a truck driver, you live quite a sedentary lifestyle, which can greatly affect your health. Also, since you are on the road most of the time, you may not have healthy food options at your disposal most of the time, and this can lead to unhealthy eating.

In 2015, The National Institute for Occupational Safety and Health conducted a survey on truck drivers' health and injury. They collected data from 1,670 long haul drivers from 32 truck stops- and the results were shocking. They discovered that over two-thirds, which is 69 percent of the drivers, were obese (defined by BMI/body mass index of 30 or higher), and 17 percent were extremely obese (defined by BMI of 40 or higher). In contrast, only 7 percent of U.S working adults are extremely obese, and only one-third of the population is obese.

Being a long-haul tracker is one of the unhealthiest jobs in America, and the worst part is the unwanted weight you gain in this line of work puts you at a high risk of developing life-threatening illnesses like diabetes and cardiovascular disease, hypertension, and sleep apnea, just to name a few. Further, studies from the Healthy Trucking Association of America show that obesity in truck drivers leads to more accidents on the road.

Those are shocking facts, and the question now is what should you do as a truck driver to ensure you are healthy and fit and that you are not putting your life in danger of diseases or accidents?

Well, that is what this guide is here for- to hold your hands and show you the way to better health and being fit. You will learn the steps you need to take now to change your diet and incorporate exercises into your lifestyle for a healthier YOU.

Table of Contents

Chapter 1: How Did You Get Here?

As a truck driver who wants to change from being unhealthy, at risk of disease, and being out of shape, you must first ask yourself how you got where you are today. Understanding the problem you are in right now is important because it shows you the wrong path you took and helps you know what needs to be done to live a healthy lifestyle.

In 2011, a 50-year-old California-based long-haul truck driver, Richard Hall, went for his first Department of Transportation medical exam. When the medical examiner looked at Hall's blood work results, he said, "You should be in a coma." Hall's blood sugar level was 392. The normal sugar level is less than 140, and a sugar level of above 200 means you have diabetes. Hall was 392, how dangerous is that!

If you think that is worse, then this next story will blow your mind.

Justin Boschee, a 27-year-old long-haul truck driver, was once instructed to switch trailers with one of his colleagues. He located his colleague and knocked on the truck door, but there was no answer. He later discovered the truck driver had diabetes and that on that day, when he knocked on his cabin, the truck driver had breathed his last.

As a trucker who is overweight and unhealthy, those two incidents could have happened to you.

But how did you get here?

Well, there is no one thing that you did to get here. What you did is a combination of things that has made it nearly impossible for you to remain fit and healthy as a truck driver.

Let me break it down for you.

The schedules that as a truck driver you keep and the nature of your job make it quite easy for you to gain weight and be obese.

First and foremost, as a truck driver, you spend most of your time on the road. It is approximated that a normal truck driver spends up to 300 days a year on the road. Now the reason you gain weight has a lot to do with how you spend those 300days; you spend them sitting down.

An average trucker spends up to 11 hours driving. When you are not driving, you are mostly seated somewhere in a restaurant eating or sleeping, which means you spend a lot of time inactive. In addition, since you do not have much time to spare for a regular gym session, you rarely get to exercise. That lifestyle is what has led you here-being overweight and leaving an unhealthy life.

Here is the deal when your body is inactive, and you are eating the typical- three meals per day- you have more energy than you need, which leads to your body converting the surplus energy into body fat. That then leads to fast weight gain, and it is the reason for your weight gain.

But inactivity is not the only thing that has landed you here; your poor feeding habits have also played a huge part in leading an unhealthy lifestyle. What is interesting, though, is the circumstances of your work influence your bad eating habits.

As a truck driver, you live in 'a box', a cabin with no kitchen, no food storage, or at least not storage that can store food for a good number of days. So, when it comes down to meals, you must rely on truck stop shops, which are the only places that, as a truck driver, you can effectively park and take a break to eat when you are on the road. Now truck stops mostly stock unhealthy fast foods like Salisbury steak, cheeseburgers, French fries, hot dogs, among others. They also offer unhealthy snacks to go, like sodas, energy bars, crisps, etc. They offer those types of food more than they stock healthy foods like fresh fruits, salads, and other healthy natural foods.

Since you cannot go to a Farmer's market and have a kitchen to cook for yourself, you must eat the unhealthy food options at your disposal, and this leads to weight gain and puts you at risk of lifestyle diseases.

Also, you are likely to engage in risky behaviors that make you prone to health risks. According to a CDC study, more than half of trucker's smoke cigarettes, as compared to only 19 percent in the general population.

The other reason you are obese has to do with your metabolism related to your circadian rhythms, sleep cycles, and accumulated sleep stress and debt.

Your schedule is nothing like the typical 9-5 job where you are in the same place. As a trucker, you make pick-ups and deliveries as you keep up with hours-of-service requirements, which get your sleep cycles and rhythms out of sync. This then slows down your metabolism and results in weight gain.

That is how you got here.

Now, why is it so crucial for you to turn your lifestyle around, lose weight and concentrate on living a healthy life?

Here are a few reasons that highlight why it is important to work on your health and fitness.

It helps you keep your job.

One of the obvious benefits of losing weight is it helps you keep your job as a trucker. As you know, the trucking profession keeps you on the road for long periods. As highlighted, this leads to weight gain and, even in some cases, obesity. Obesity puts your body at risk of contracting a host of health diseases such as stroke, back pain, cancer, heart disease, high blood pressure, and type 2 diabetes, among others.

Now you might not know this, but the conditions above are not just deadly but can also affect your livelihood. This is because The Federal Motor Safety Commission conducts regular medical evaluations on all truckers.

Suppose you undergo an evaluation and are found with a high health risk like having high blood pressure. In that case, you are disqualified from receiving your commercial driver's license, or you will lose your driving license, which will automatically take away your livelihood. The government believes such conditions impair your driving ability- which is true.

When you lose weight and live a healthier lifestyle, you decrease your health risk, which enables you to keep your livelihood.

Reduce your risk of life-threatening diseases.

The biggest disadvantage of the unhealthy lifestyle you are leading right now is that it increases your risk of developing life-threatening conditions like heart disease, stroke, type 2 diabetes, cancer, and blood pressure. These conditions are extremely dangerous to your health. As you saw earlier in Justin Boschee's story, these conditions do not just make your life miserable but can also lead to death.

When you start watching what you eat and incorporate workouts in your life, you significantly reduce your risk of suffering from life-threatening conditions.

Here is a list of some obese-related chronic diseases and how losing weight prevents you from them.

Cancer

When you are obese or overweight, your chances of developing cancers such as cancers of the stomach, pancreas, gallbladder, kidney, liver, rectum, and colon increases immensely.

This is because when gaining weight, you consume a lot of food, which results in high levels of glucose in your body and high levels of insulin (the media that is used to transport glucose to your cells). An extended period of this spike creates the perfect environment for the growth of tumors, which can be cancerous.

When working on losing weight, you reduce your food intake. This will, in turn, lead to lower glucose levels because you are not taking as much food; thus, reducing your risk of getting cancer.

High blood pressure

When you gain weight, what typically happens is your body slowly starts to put some extra strain on how your heart pumps blood. When this goes on for an extended period, it develops into high blood pressure, a major risk factor of chronic conditions like heart attack and stroke.

When you lose weight, even by as little as 10 pounds, you can lower your blood pressure.

Type 2 diabetes

If you look at people who have diabetes, you will realize that 90 percent are overweight or obese.

Why.

Because weight gain is a major risk factor for diabetes, when you are overweight, you are likely eating more foods high in carbohydrates, which, when broken down, increases glucose levels. Pancreas then releases insulin to help with the transportation of the glucose to the cells, with the extra glucose being converted to glycogen and fat. As you take foods high in carbohydrates, there is a greater demand for insulin to manage glucose levels. Over time, the pancreas may be unable to keep up since you need more and more insulin, which can lead to insulin resistance, a precursor to type 2 diabetes.

Losing weight, especially by adopting a low carb diet, helps prevent chances of diabetes since there will be less glucose and the demand for insulin will reduce; thus, avoiding instances of insulin resistance.

Increased Energy levels

It takes a fair amount of energy and concentration to drive for long periods. When you are overweight, the extra weight tends to take a toll on your body, and you find yourself feeling fatigued, or you start experiencing chronic pain in your joints, knees, back, and hips. This affects your concentration and efficiency at work.

Now the advantage of losing weight is that it helps you reverse this situation. One of the first things you will notice when you lose weight is high energy levels. This is so because you use minimal energy in your day-to-day activity when you are carrying fewer pounds. Weight loss also tends to enhance your oxygen efficiency, meaning you will no longer find yourself out of breath when doing simple chores that do not require too much energy.

Better Sleep

As someone who spends 11 hours or more on the road, you need as much rest as you can get. When you are overweight and unhealthy, it sometimes becomes challenging to get this rest because of weight-related conditions like snoring and sleep apnea that affect your sleep quality. When you adopt a healthy lifestyle and lose weight, you lose the excess weight around your neck, which plays a role in sleep apnea. So, once you shed that, your night rest will improve, helping you get the rest you deserve.

You now must be thinking those are tremendous benefits and at the same time asking yourself how you can be able to achieve and maintain a healthy and fit lifestyle.

Well, there are unique ways you can use to stay healthy and in shape while you are on the road -which will be explained further in the subsequent chapters starting with the next chapter, which is going to focus on educating you on how to change your lifestyle to a healthy one through diet.

Chapter 2: Healthy Diets for Weight Loss

As you now know, driving a truck can easily lead to obesity. As shocking as this may be, being overweight and at risk of chronic disease is normal to truck drivers. It is so normal that people get shocked when they see a truck driver who is not overweight or obese and rarely believe that he/she is a truck driver.

Now, this is mostly because of what you eat.

Unfortunately, truck driving is one of those jobs where most people eat the unhealthiest foods. You most likely survive on junk foods in the name of 'energy foods.' The sad part is that you never really get as much energy, and you may experience energy spikes and lows, making you opt for more food for that dose of energy, and the cycle continues.

Anyway, I do understand that being healthy while on the road can be a huge challenge.

And the problem is not that there are not good food options on the road. The problem is that you are bombarded with a lot of tempting easy to go, high calories foods that look yummy and delicious- but are downright unhealthy.

The good news is that you can change this. You can go from being obese, unhealthy, and suffering or at risk of suffering from a wide range of diseases to a healthy lean person.

But how do you get here?

Well, there is not really one diet but rather a combination of diets that are great and adopting healthy eating habits that will enable you to stay healthy and keep fit.

This chapter will focus on two of the best diets that will help you stay fit and maintain a healthy lifestyle on the road.

Let us start with the first diet:

The Keto Diet

Following the keto diet is an effective and efficient way to lose weight, get fit, and live a healthier life. So, what exactly is the ketogenic diet? How can you lose weight while on this diet and is it possible to follow this diet while on the road?

Let me answer these questions:

In a nutshell, the ketogenic diet entails eating foods low in carbohydrates, having moderate protein, and high in fats. This diet basically requires you to eliminate sugar-rich foods and all carbs from grains like crackers, pasta, and bread and get your carbohydrates from fruits and vegetables while getting more of your calories from fats.

This diet's main aim is to help you reach the metabolic state of ketosis where your body changes its metabolism from burning carbohydrates for energy to burning fats for energy.

So, how does this diet help you lose weight? To understand that, you need to know how your body works and the effects it creates and how ketosis works, and its effects on your body.

The Conventional diet

When you follow a conventional diet, which is generally high in carbs, moderate or high in protein, and low in fats- your body breaks down the three macronutrients above in search of energy. Since carbohydrates are the simplest macronutrients to breakdown and absorb, your body breaks them down first into glucose, which it immediately uses as energy. It then breaks down fats into fatty acids, which it stores in your fat stores as a secondary energy source that your body can use when it is starved of its number one energy source, glucose. Proteins are then broken down into amino acids, which are used in your muscles.

So why does the keto diet want to discourage your body from burning carbohydrates for energy? This is because all that you are today -obese and overweight - and what you might be going through or at risk of going through-illnesses like diabetes, cancer, and high blood pressure are all engineered by this process of your body burning carbohydrates for energy.

Here is how.

Two things happen when your body burns carbohydrates for energy.

It turns your body into a fat-storing machine. As you saw earlier, when you eat a meal, your body breaks down carbohydrates to glucose for energy while converting any extra glucose to glycogen and fats to use as energy when you are starved. But unlike the caveman days where starving was a real possibility, today, starving is a rare thing.

In fact, when last did you starve, and by this, I mean going for more than 15 hours without food? Probably never.

What this means is that when following a conventional diet, your body continually stores fats that you never use. These fats pile up in your body and make you overweight and obese, and all this is made possible by insulin.

Insulin is a hormone produced by your pancreas for the sole reason of it controlling your blood sugar. When you eat carbohydrate-rich food, your body will produce insulin, which transports glucose into your cells to be used as energy, and any excess, as mentioned, is converted to fat for storage.

Insulin plays a part in affecting your health. When you follow a conventional diet, insulin becomes ever-present in your body. While this might sound like a good thing because it helps in energy supply, it is not.

And that's because high levels of insulin in your body have been promoting some of the problems you have been going through. When insulin is high in your body, fat cannot be broken down for energy. Also, high insulin levels lead to lower blood sugar levels within a short time as insulin does its job of regulating blood sugar, leading to cravings owing to the sudden low in energy. By doing so, it destabilizes your energy levels.

High insulin levels can also lead to diabetes, where your cells stop responding to insulin, which inhibits them from receiving glucose to use as energy. A situation that becomes fatal to your body because high glucose levels in your bloodstream can damage your blood vessels. Now you understand why you need to change your eating habits.

Now, here is why ketosis works and why it is the best diet for you to follow if you are to be healthy and fit again:

While following the keto diet, your macronutrient intake ratio is 75 percent fat, 5 percent carbohydrates, and 20 percent protein. This means 5 percent of calories in your meal should come from carbohydrates, 20 percent from protein, and 75 percent from fats. So, how does this make you healthy and lean?

It does that by helping you reach the metabolic state of ketosis.

When you eat a high-fat, low-carb meal, your body does not have access to its preferred source of energy, glucose and so what it does is it flips your metabolism pathway and starts burning fats for energy. At first, your body will burn your ingested fats into ketones, which it uses as fuel. However, once that is done, it moves to your fat storages (you remember those that were always being filled up by a high carb diet for later use?) and breaks them down into fatty acids and glycerol, which are used as fuel for your body.

In short, your body turns into a fat burning machine that does not only turn your fat gaining process into a fat-losing process, helping you lose weight but also minimizing the production of insulin, eliminating fat storage, cravings, and disease like type 2 diabetes.

So how do you get started with this effective diet for weight loss?

Let us start with the foods that you need to avoid.

Foods to avoid.

The keto diet is a low carb diet; therefore, most foods you need to avoid are those high in carbs. You want to try your best and limit the supply of glucose in your body so that your body can continue being a fat-burning machine.

Here is a list of foods you should eliminate from your diet:

- Grains and grain products like cereals, pasta, and rice

- Legumes like chickpeas, lentils, beans, and peas

- Tubers and root vegetables like parsnips, sweet potatoes, and potatoes

- Fruits high in sugar like banana, mangoes, watermelon, pineapple, etc

- Sugary foods, which include candy, ice cream, cake, soda, and others.

- Sugar-free diet foods like desserts, sweeteners, pudding, syrups, and sugar-free candies

- Alcoholic drinks like liquor, wine, and beer, which your body concentrates on burning for energy once ingested.

- Unhealthy fats like mayonnaise and processed oils like vegetable oils

- Sauces with sugar like ketchup, teriyaki sauce, honey, mustard, and barbecue sauce

Foods to eat.

Your foods should be high in fat and low in carbohydrates. Let us look at some of the foods you can eat:

- Low carb condiments like spices, herbs, salt, and pepper

- Low carb vegetables like peppers, onions, leafy green vegetables

- Healthy low-carb oils like avocado oil, coconut oil, and extra virgin olive oil

- Seeds and nuts such as chia seeds, pumpkin seeds, flaxseeds, walnuts, and almonds

- Fruits such as strawberries, blackberries, blueberries, olives, and avocados

- Cheeses like mozzarella, cream, cheddar, and blue

- Heavy cream and butter

- Eggs

- Fatty fish like mackerel, tuna, trout, and salmon

- Healthy snacks: As a truck driver, you might get hungry between meals and need a bite. Instead of snacking on unhealthy food, you can snack on the following healthy snacks.

    ✓ Small portions of your left-over meals

    ✓ Guacamole

    ✓ Cheese with strawberries

    ✓ Nuts and seeds

    ✓ Boiled eggs

✓ Beef jerky

✓ Fat bombs

Now when it comes down to it, there are two ways you can go about following the keto diet.

The first one is preparing keto meals that you can eat for one week on the road. With this method, you will have to set aside 4-5 hours every week to do some shopping and prepare meals for the whole week.

Here is a list of healthy meals that you can prepare once and enjoy all week on the road.

For breakfast, you can prepare,

- Keto breakfast scramble with Cajun sausage

- Milkshake- flavored protein shakes.

- Keto blueberry muffins

- Avocado scramble

- Keto egg cups

For lunch, you can prepare,

- Spinach salmon burgers

- Keto Taco cheeseburgers

- Mediterranean salad.

- Zoodle salad with peanut and ginger

- Keto meatballs

For dinner, you can prepare,

- Keto pork chops with sweet chili

- Buffalo chicken salad.

- Creamy ham and broccoli casserole

- Jalapeno shrimp veggie bakes.

It is easy, really, if you are willing to put in the work and achieve good health. You just need to make the meals mentioned above before leaving for the week and pack them in a fridge or a cooler. Then once ready to eat, take each one out and microwave. If the meals are kept refrigerated, they should serve you a good number of days.

If this is not a possible solution for you, you can still follow a keto diet by eating out in restaurants, including fast-food restaurants. All you must do is to be creative and eat keto-friendly meals.

For instance, you can:

- Eat healthy salads seasoned with pepper and salt with shrimp, steak, chicken, and opt for olive oil as your dressing.

- Ask for taco salads and burrito bowls that contain veggies, cheese, guacamole, and meats minus the taco shell, tortillas, and chips.

- Ask for bunless sandwiches and burgers minus fries, breading, sauces, and sweet condiments.

- For breakfast, you can opt for eggs, berry smoothies without added sugar, some bacon, and sausages.

- You can also carry healthy keto snacks such as nuts and seeds like almonds, walnuts, pumpkin seeds, chia seeds.

Any of the above meals will have you following a keto diet and feeling satisfied as you gradually lose weight and betters your health.

The fantastic thing about the keto diet is the diet is high in fat, which is denser and provides more energy. Therefore, you will feel fuller for longer, have more energy, and have better concentration because you will not be experiencing the energy spikes and lows.

That said, you need to check with your doctor before starting the diet to ensure that you do not have any underlying conditions that could worsen by adopting the keto diet.

Another great way you can lose weight and live a healthier lifestyle is by practicing intermittent fasting.

Intermittent Fasting

If you have been paying close attention to the health and fitness trends lately, you have probably come across the words intermittent fasting. Intermittent fasting is one of the most popular eating plans. So popular is intermittent fasting that many celebrities swear by it, including Kourtney Kardashian, Scarlett Johansson, Vanessa Hodgens, and Mindy Kaling, to name a few.

Intermittent fasting has been a revolution but not just in the general population but in the trucking industry. It has immensely helped long haul truck drivers get fit and live healthy lives despite them sitting down driving for more than 10 hours a day. Here are truckers that have lost weight through following intermittent fasting.

In an interview with men's health magazine, Carlos Soto told the magazine that he had lost 30 pounds by following intermittent fasting and doing a little exercise.

A truck driver known as James, who has a YouTube channel named James Views, started practicing intermittent fasting. When James started, he weighed 305 pounds, and after 30 days of intermittent fasting, he had lost 50 pounds weighing 255.

A truck driver known as King was featured on a YouTube channel called a healthy Alternative, explained how he lost 140 pounds with intermittent fasting.

As you can see, this diet is effective, and it can be effective for you too. But what is intermittent fasting, where did it come from, how does it work, and how can you get started with it?

Well, this chapter is going to explain all that, starting with what intermittent fasting is.

Intermittent fasting is not a diet per se but more of an eating pattern where you cycle between eating and fasting. In other words, intermittent fasting entails scheduling your meals to allow you to have feasting times and fasting times.

One of the best things about this eating pattern is unlike other diets; it does not tell you what to eat and how much to eat, rather when you should eat.

But isn't that starvation?

The answer is no. Fasting is vastly different from starvation. Starvation is when you involuntary do not eat because of lack of food for long periods. This usually leads to severe suffering or death. On the flip side, fasting is when you have access to food, but you choose not to eat for a specific period.

So, where did this pattern of eating come from?

This might come as a surprise to you, but intermittent fasting is an ancient way of eating. Fasting has been practiced throughout evolution from ancient cultures and religions on Earth. It was our original way of eating.

So, it is true what Marie Antoinette once said, 'There is nothing new, except what has been forgotten.'

Centuries ago, our forefathers, unlike us, did not have refrigerators, supermarkets, or food all year round. They were hunters and gatherers who depended on what they caught in the wild or gathered for food. Now many times, our ancestors could not find food, which forced them to go for hours or even days without food.

As a result, we evolved to that system, and our bodies adapted, and fasting became natural to us. In fact, our bodies function better when we go for extended periods without food. It is why our forefathers did not suffer from some of the conditions we suffer from today, like obesity, diabetes, cancer, stroke, and heart attacks, to name but a few.

Therefore, following intermittent fasting is going back to the way humans are designed to eat.

But why would you adopt intermittent fasting? Why would you go back and start eating in a way that your forefathers ate?

Well, there are a couple of reasons why it is worth your while to start practicing intermittent fasting.

First, it is a great way to get lean without following a crazy diet that cuts your calories down to a point that it becomes unnatural for you to stick to the diet.

Secondly and perhaps the most important is this way of eating helps you lose weight. Finally, it is an easy eating strategy that we are designed for, which means it is simple enough for you to do it and impactful enough for it to make a difference in your health and fitness.

To understand all that, you need to know how intermittent fasting works.

As mentioned earlier, intermittent fasting enables you to enjoy several benefits, including weight loss, being lean, and reduced risk of suffering from chronic disease. But how does it do it. To understand that you will need to understand the fed state, post absorptive state and fasted state.

Fed state

The fed state is the period during which your body is digesting as well as absorbing food. The fed state typically starts when you start eating and lasts for 3-5 hours after that. During this time, it absorbs and digests the foods you have been eating. When you are in this state, your body cannot burn fat because your insulin is high, meaning your body is using glucose for energy.

Post-absorptive state

Five hours after you eat, your body crosses over to the post absorption state. In this state, your body does not process any meal. This state normally lasts until 8 to 12 hours after you eat your last meal.

Fasted state

Eight to twelve hours after your last meal, your body enters the fasted state. In this state, all the food you ate has been used up, and you have no active energy left. So, what your body does is it moves to your second energy source, which is stored fat and starts to burn them for energy. Do you remember the metabolic state of ketosis?

That is the state that you get into in this stage. As you now know, ketosis allows you to enjoy several benefits, including weight loss, prevention of cancer, blood pressure, type 2 diabetes, increased energy, and many more.

Basically, with intermittent fasting, you go without food for more than 12 hours (that you do not do with the conventional way of eating), getting you into the beneficial state of ketosis where your body starts burning fat for energy, which then leads to weight loss.

This might come as a surprise to you, but intermittent fasting is not a new thing to you. You might have done it a couple of times in your life, but you did not know it was called intermittent fasting.

Have you ever eaten dinner early, let us say at 8 p.m., then you went to bed late, like midnight, and woke up the next morning at 11 a.m. and had your breakfast at around 11:30 a.m.? If you have ever done this, then you have done intermittent fasting. In fact, that day you fasted for 15 hours 30 minutes. Plus, every night you sleep two hours after your last meal, you fast for 10-12 hours. So intermittent fasting is not a new thing in your life; it is just something that makes you prolong the fast you already were doing in your life to benefit your fitness and health.

There are different approaches that you can take to start intermittent fasting. All these approaches you are about to read are effective and can help you stay fit, healthy and lose weight. That said, as an individual, there is one that will suit you better. I will highlight five of the most common intermittent fasting protocols, and you can choose one that is best suited to you.

The 16:8 Method

If you want to lose body fat while building some muscles, you should follow this intermittent fasting plan.

The 16/8 method is one of the easiest intermittent fasting methods. This method requires you to fast every day for 14-16 hours and then have an eating window of 8-10 hours. It is recommended that women fast for 14 hours because they seem to do better with shorter fasts, and men do better with more extended fasts like the 16 hour fast.

During the feeding window, you can have 2-3 meals. Here you can eat anything you like; however, remember that as a truck driver driving for long distances, you need your energy. Therefore, it is best to opt for nutrient-dense meals that will keep you full. Also, since you are not eating too many meals, you must make the few meals you take count by eating highly balanced meals to ensure that you get all the nutrients your body needs.

You may probably be thinking about how you can fast 14-16 hours. Well, it is not as hard as you think.

It is as simple as not eating anything after your dinner and then having a late breakfast.

For example, if you usually finish your dinner at 8 p.m., go to bed at 10 p.m. and take breakfast at 8 a.m., it means you have naturally been fasting for 12 hours. So, this method will just require you to move your breakfast ahead by 4 hours to have it at noon if you are a man and move it by 2hours to have it at 10 a.m. if you are a woman.

It is as easy as that. In case you find 8 a.m. to 12 noon or 10 a.m. fast hard for you, you can drink non-caloric beverages like coffee and water. They will help reduce your cravings and hunger without interfering with your metabolism process of burning fat for energy.

The 5:2 Method

This is one of the easiest intermittent fasting methods. As a beginner, it is one of the best methods you can start with.

The idea with the 5:2 method is simple. Eat normally for five days. For instance, if you eat three meals per day and a snack in between, continue with that schedule for five days, and then for two days, eat only 500 calories if you are a woman and 600 calories if you are a man a day.

The two fasting days should be between feasting days. For instance, if Monday is a fasting day, Tuesday should be a feasting day, then Wednesday a fasting day, and you can then eat normally until Monday when you go back to fasting.

This method is for you if you feel like fasting every day is too much for you. Although you do not lose so much weight on this method, it helps you have a smooth transition into fasting, which you can use as a steppingstone to other more demanding fasting methods.

The Warrior Diet

If you are a trucker who likes following rules and want a method that will help you get fit and lose weight faster, then the warrior diet is for you.

The warrior diet emphasizes 'under-eating'.

So, how does it work?

This method mimics the life of real warriors who train for almost the whole day and only eat one large meal.

With this intermittent fasting method, you fast for 20 hours every day and only eat one large meal at night. It is advisable to eat at night so that you can be in sync with your circadian rhythms by feeding your body the nutrients it needs.

While fasting for 20 hours is challenging, the good news is that during the 20-hour fast, you can eat a few servings of vegetables, raw fruits, and boiled eggs. The idea is to keep your calories intake extremely low.

In the 4-hour feasting window, you must eat foods with nutrients that help your body repair and grow. Immediately, it is time to eat; you should start with eating veggies. If you are still hungry, eat some protein, then fats, and finally carbohydrates if you still feel hungry. That order will help you get the best out of this method.

Alternate Day Fasting

This approach is like the 5:2 method, with the only difference being that instead of fasting for two days in a week, you fast every other day. This means you alternate your week between feasting days and fasting days. So, how does it work?

The idea here is for you to eat normally one day and eat little the next day. Rinse and repeat until the end of the week. For example, on the fasting day, eat one-fifth of your normal calorie intake if you are a man and one fourth if you are a woman. In this case, you can eat normally on Monday, fast on Tuesday, eat as you typically do on Wednesday, and so forth.

This approach was popularized was developed by a nutrition professor called Krista Varady at the University of Illinois in Chicago, specifically for weight loss.

This diet allows you to take non-caloric drinks like water or coffee to help you fight off hunger and cravings to cope with the low-calorie days. In case you do regular workouts, you may find it challenging to perform high-intensity exercises. What you need to do is to schedule easy and low intense workouts on your low days.

Your food selection is also not restricted, but it is advisable for you to eat a healthy meal. Dr. Varady and his colleagues did a study they published in Nutrition Journal where they discovered this approach was highly effective in helping obese adults lose weight.

Eat Stop Eat

Brad Pilon started the Eat Stop Eat method. This method entails fasting for 24 hours once or two times a week, then eating as you normally would during the remaining 5 days of the week.

A good way to practice eat stop eat is for example, if your last meal of the day was at 8 p.m., you should not eat anything for 24 hours until the following day at 8 p.m.

As always, ensure that you eat responsibly to nourish your body and to avoid instances of unnecessary snacking.

This method is suitable once you get used to intermittent fasting because fasting for 24 hours is quite intense if you are a beginner.

Those are the five main intermittent fasting methods you can use to lose weight, get fit and live a healthy lifestyle.

I would advise you to try out each of the five methods and see which one works best for you and your needs. That said, fasting, especially for a newbie like you, could be challenging. It can take a toll on your body if you go 'cold turkey,' and you might never want to experience it again- and we do not want that.

Therefore, the best way to go about trying out the different intermittent fasting methods is to ease into fasting. This means that you do not do the whole fast when you start; instead, start with few minutes of fasting and increase that number until you can do the whole fast.

If we take the 16:8 method as an example, if your schedule is to eat your dinner at 8 p.m. and take breakfast at 7 a.m., it means you fast every day for 11 hours. So, what you can do when you start is to push your breakfast by 30 minutes.

So, take your breakfast at 7:30 a.m. Do that for three days, then add another half hour and give your body three days to adjust. Repeat until you can finally do the whole 16 hours fast.

If you ever feel hungry when fasting, have some non-caloric drinks, and the best one is water. You could also have unsweetened tea and coffee, which will reduce your cravings and hunger; thus, enabling you to manage your fasting better.

You could opt to adapt either the ketogenic diet or intermittent fasting or you could combine them for effective weight loss. Many people have had great success practicing intermittent fasting and adapting the ketogenic diet.

In addition to changing your diet, you also need to increase your activity levels to become fit. The next chapter will focus on this:

Chapter 3: Workouts for Better Health

The other effective way to stay fit is to work out on the road. As a long-haul truck driver, you know how demanding your job can be. You are seated driving for long hours and only have a few hours to sleep. Therefore, it is not surprising to sometimes be sedentary for almost over 20 hours per day, and this is what makes you think being on the road for long hours means you cannot have time to stay in shape and healthy. But you are mistaken.

You can exercise on the road and manage to lose weight, maintain your weight, stay fit, and be healthy. You must be creative and be determined and consistent to achieve your goals.

According to the American Heart Association, to be healthy and fit you need to get at least 30 minutes of moderately intense exercise five days a week. Your first goal should be to manage the 30 minutes of moderately intense exercise for five days in a week as a truck driver.

But how are you supposed to do that? The best way to go about it is by spreading the 30 minutes exercise into 2-3 small sessions in a day. But how do you get those free 10- 20- minute sessions for exercising in a line of work that keeps you busy almost all day?

Well, you must be creative and start finding ways to use whatever little time you have to exercise and get in shape. Here are scenarios that you can take advantage of and sneak some exercises.

You can take some minutes to exercise immediately you wake up in the morning.

You can use a few minutes of your lunch break to exercise-preferably before having your lunch.

Use that 10-20 free minutes that you have at a rest shop.

Grab the few minutes you have when waiting for your truck to be loaded up or unloaded.

If you take your truck to be checked out by a mechanic on the road, you can use that time to exercise.

You can also use the free minutes you get when you fuel your truck to sneak some exercises.

When it comes down to the exercise you should do, the idea is to have a workout program that ensures you exercise every part of your body. Here are some easy workouts you can carry out for different parts of your body.

To do these exercises, though, you will need a few pieces of equipment you can use while on your truck to make your workouts more effective and comfortable.

Some of these things include:

- Yoga mat

- Resistance band

- Kettle bell

- Dumbbells

Here are the groups of exercises.

Warm-ups

It is crucial to do some warm-up exercises before doing any of the exercises we will look at later in the book.

Here are a few good warm-up exercises that will get your heart rate up.

Jogging

Jogging around your truck is an excellent way to get your heart rate up, and it does not strain any of your joints.

Jumping jacks

Jumping jacks is another brilliant exercise that can get your heart rate up. It is best to do jumping jacks for 1-2 minutes. This will awaken your body and get your blood flowing well, but you must raise your arms up above your head if you are to get the best out of it.

How to do them:

Step 1: Start by standing upright with your legs together. Place your arms at your sides.

Step 2: Slowly bend your knees and jump into the air.

Step 3: As you jump, stretch your arms out over your head and spread your legs apart- shoulder width.

Step 4: Go back to the starting position. Repeat.

Push-ups

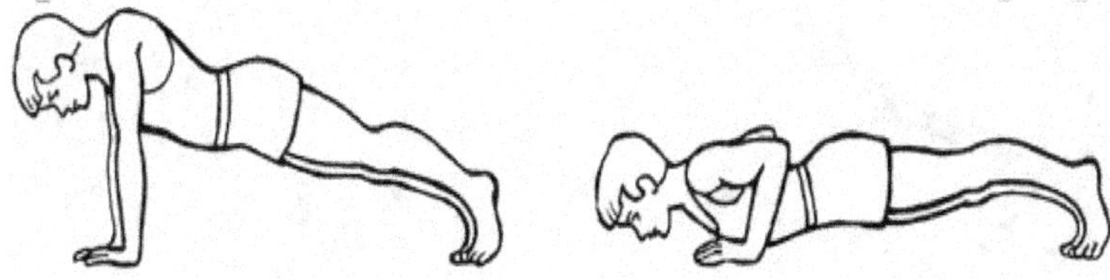

Push-ups are good for working out your upper body, glutes, and core.

How to do them

Step 1: Be on all fours, move your hands apart- slightly wider than your shoulders.

Step 2: Straighten your legs and arms.

Step 3: Slowly lower your body until your chest is almost touching the floor. Pause for a few seconds, and then push you back up. Repeat.

Leg Swings

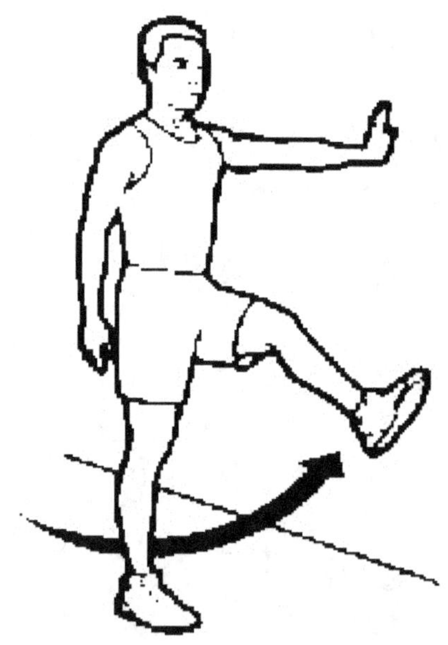

How to do them:

Step 1: Start by standing on one foot. As a beginner, you can stand next to your truck and hold the truck for support with one hand.

Step 2: Stand upright and tighten your core.

Step 3: Start swinging your leg forward and backward like a pendulum. Start slow and gather momentum to achieve a full range of motion.

Step 4: Do the same with the other leg.

Arm Circles

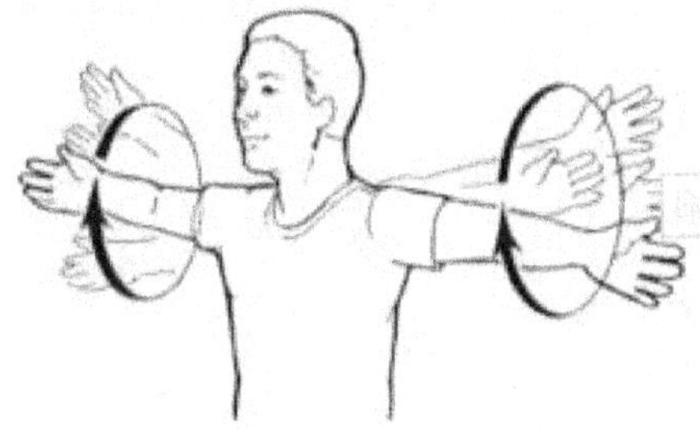

How to do them:

Step 1: Start by standing with your feet shoulder-width apart and stretch your arms parallel to the floor.

Step 2: Slowly start circling your arms forward in small, reserved motions and then gradually increase the motion and make the circles bigger until you start feeling a stretch on your triceps.

Step 3: Switch the direction of the circles after 15-25 seconds and repeat.

Core Exercise

Here are a couple of core exercises you can do:

Straight-arm plank

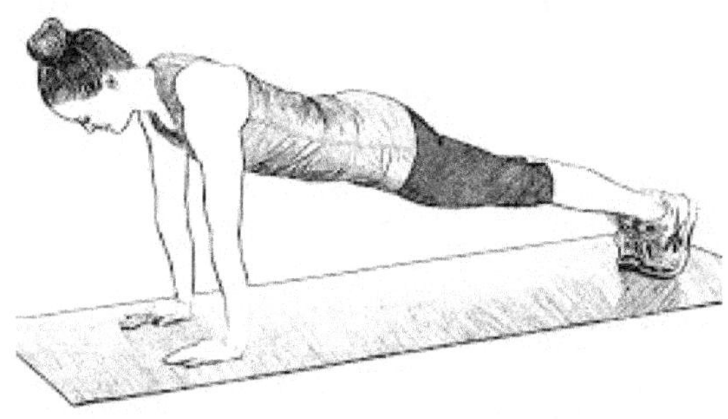

The straight-arm plank helps to build your deep inner core muscles and improve your posterior muscles' flexibility.

How to do them:

Step 1: Lie down on the ground with your hands placed at shoulder width.

Step 2: Press down firmly and lift your body. Your hands should support your body weight, and your back must be straight. This is the plank position.

Step 3: Stay in that position for about a minute. Repeat according to the set required.

Forearm Plank

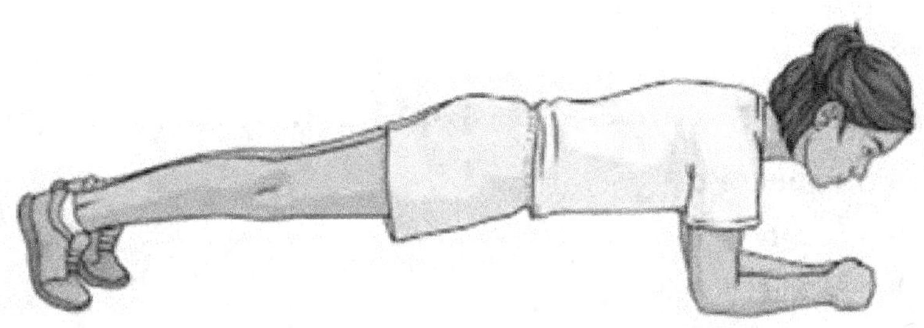

This type of plank concentrates on increasing the stability of your shoulders and aims at your abdominal muscles.

How to do it:

Step 1: Get into a plank position.

Step 2: Bend your elbows to get into a position where your elbows and toes are supporting your body weight.

Step 3: Make your hands into fists. Make sure your back is straight and face the floor. Stay in that position for 1-2 minutes.

Basic Crunches

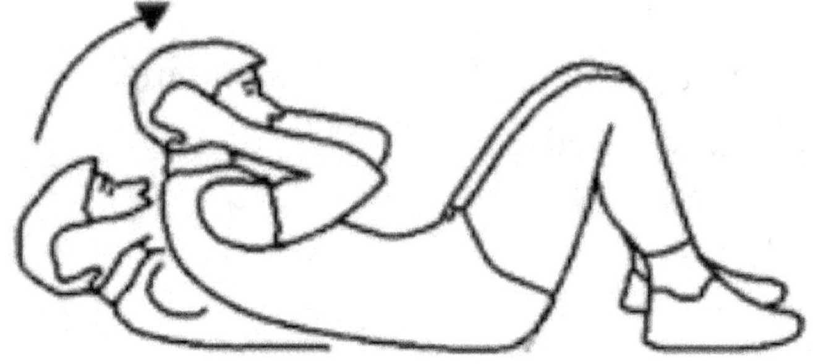

Crunches are good core exercises, and they usually train your abdominal muscles.

How to do them:

Step 1: Lie down flat on your back on your yoga mat.

Step 2: Bend your knees and plant your feet on the floor, hip-width apart.

Step 3: Place your arms right across your chest. Inhale as you contract your abs.

Step 4: Exhale and follow that up with lifting your upper body. Your abs should raise your torso towards your knees. Your neck and head should be relaxed.

Step 5: Inhale and go back to your starting position. Repeat as required.

Trunk Twist

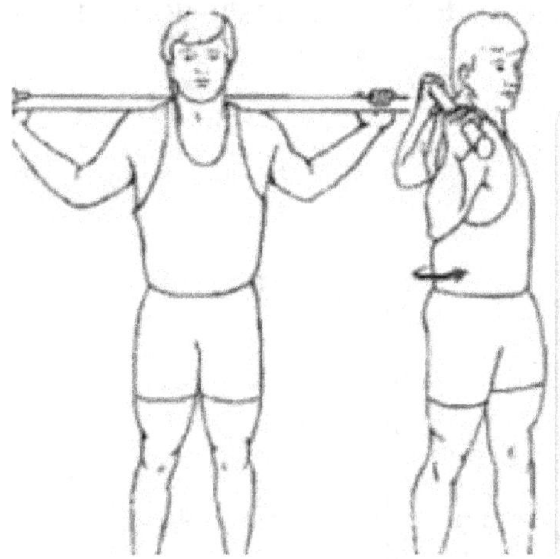

This exercise is good for stretching your back, spine, and upper torso muscles.

How to do it:

Step 1: Start by looping the resistance band through the truck's door handle.

Step 2: With the resistance band at chest- height and your legs wider than shoulder-width apart, grab the resistance band handles and then twist in the opposite direction to your door handle. If it is on your right, twist to the left while flexing your core and vice versa.

Chest and Back Exercises

You will need a resistance band to do the chest and back exercises I will highlight here. What you need to do is to loop your resistance band through the door handle of your truck and do the following exercises.

Chest fly's

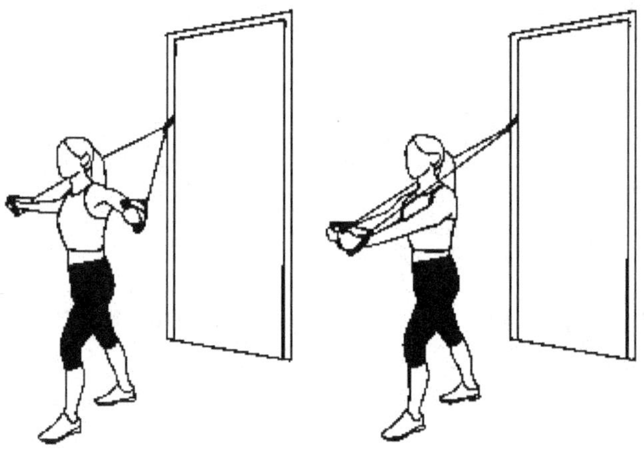

This is a good warm-up exercise for your chest.

Step 1: Hold the resistance band on your hands and stand far enough to create some tension in the bands.

Step 2: Slowly take the resistance band apart, hold for a few seconds and bring them back together in front of your chest in a kind of hugging motion. Go to the starting position and repeat.

Chest Press

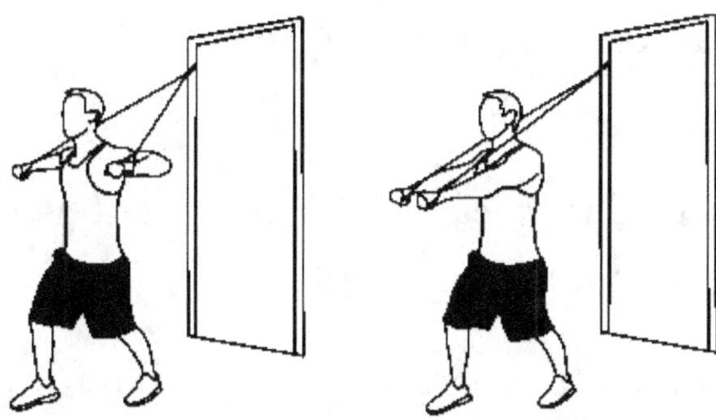

How to do it:

Step 1: With your resistance band looped through the truck's door handle, push the resistance band handles away from your body using an upward angle. Hold for a few seconds.

Step 2: Return to your starting position and repeat.

Squat Rows

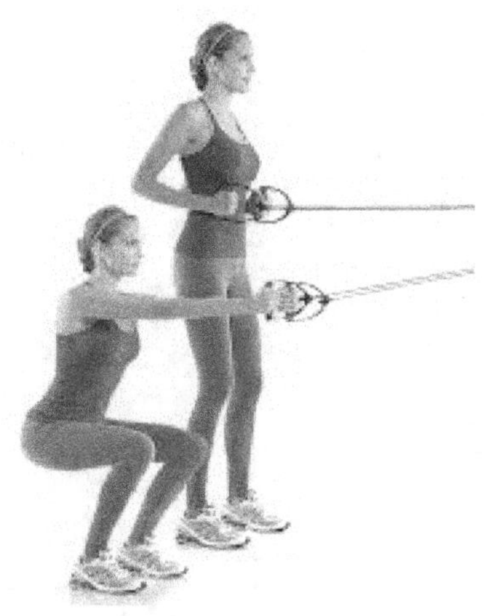

How to do it:

Step 1: Get into a squatting position while holding the resistance band.

Step 2: Pull your shoulders back and lift your chest as you pull the resistance band towards your waist.

Step 3: Hold the position for a few seconds, then go back to your starting position and repeat.

Leg Exercises

The first two exercises that you are going to do are squats. Squats are great exercises because they work your whole lower body, including your calves, hamstrings, glutes, core, and quads- and all that in just one move. Let us check out the two squats you can do:

Goblet Squats

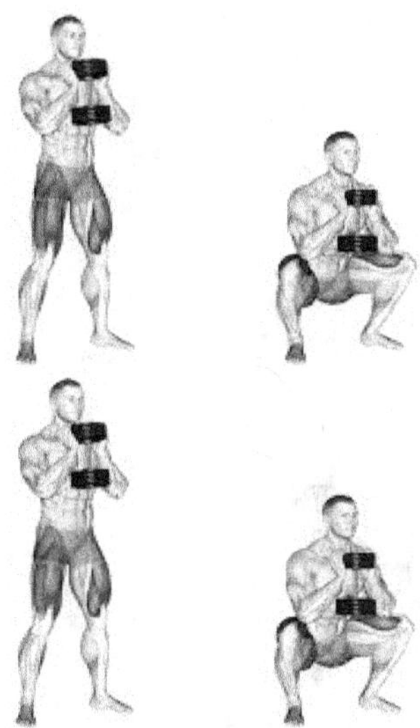

How to do them:

Step 1: Start by standing upright with your feet slightly wider than hip-distance apart. Your toes should be angled slightly outwards.

Step 2: Take a weight, whether a 3-liter bottle with handles on the side or a kettle bell and hold that with both your hands at your chest.

Step 3: Slowly bend your knees to get into a squatting position, hold and go back to the starting position.

You can start with a lighter kettle bell and work your way to a heavy one.

Front Squats

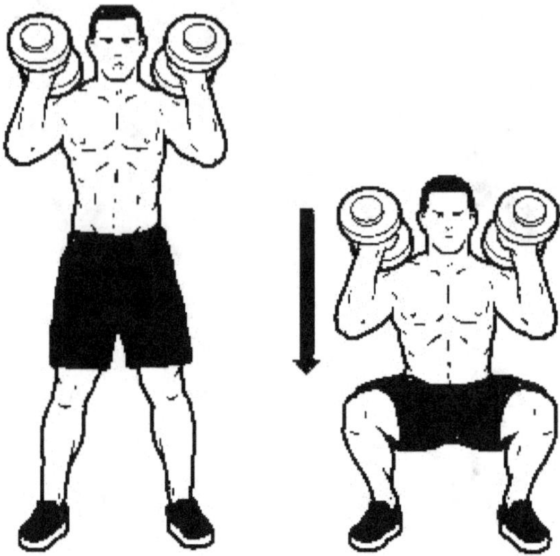

You can do front squats with kettle bells or dumbbells.

Step 1: Stand upright and place the dumbbells vertically on your shoulders.

Step 2: Bend your knees to get to a squat position, hold and get back up. Repeat as required.

Decline Lunges

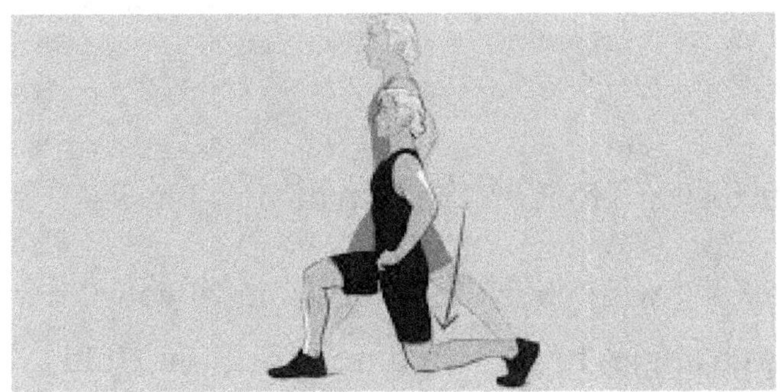

How to do them:

Step 1: Start by placing your back foot on the step of your truck.

Step 2: Move forward with your other leg until your knee reaches a 90- degree angle to lunge down. Hold for a few minutes, switch to the other leg, and repeat.

Incline Lunges

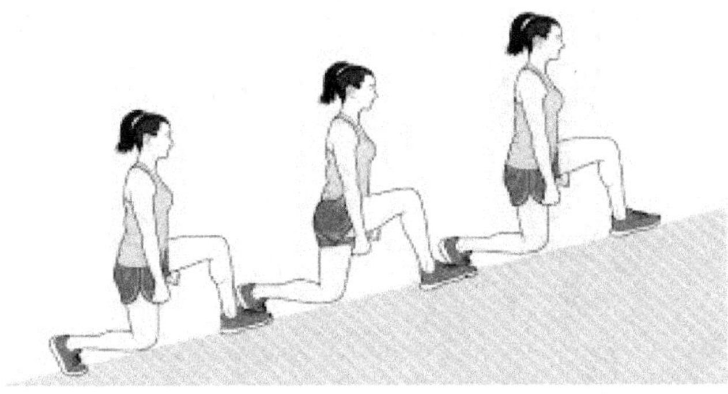

Incline lunges concentrate on your glutes while also working your hamstrings.

How to do them:

Step 1: Place your forward foot on the step of your truck.

Step 2: Hop backward with your other leg up until your knee reaches a 90-degree angle- to get to a lunge position. Hold on to that position for a few minutes and repeat for the other leg.

Arm Exercises

Most likely, your arms get sore and stiff from all the driving you do, and for that, you need to exercise your arms.

Here are a few arm exercises you can do.

Bicep Curls

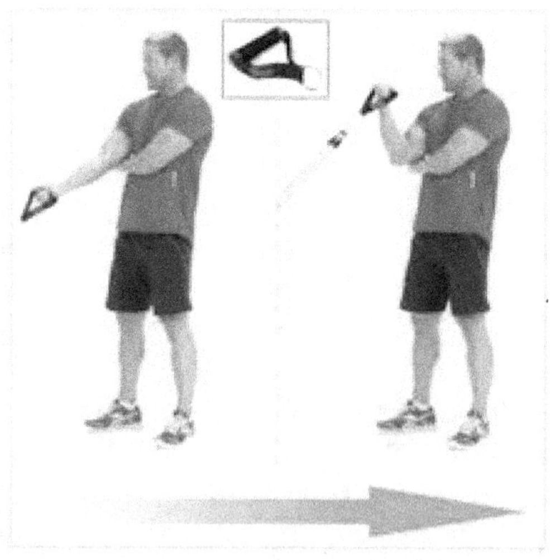

How to do them:

Step 1: Start by looping your resistance band in the door handle.

Step 2: Stand upright facing your truck door. Hold the resistance band using one hand and use your other hand to support this hand.

Step 3: Raise the band until your arm is vertical. Wait for a few seconds and return to the original position and repeat.

Preacher's Curls

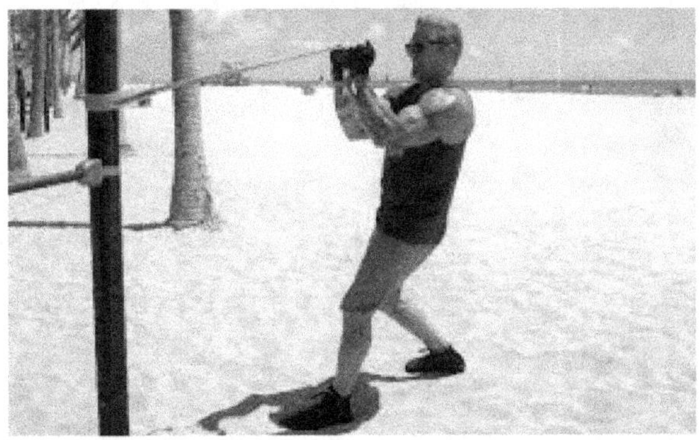

How to do them:

Step 1: With your resistance band looping through your truck door handle, take some steps back while holding the resistance band.

Step 2: Pull the band towards your chest; your movement should be focused on your biceps. Go back to the starting position and repeat.

Triceps Extensions

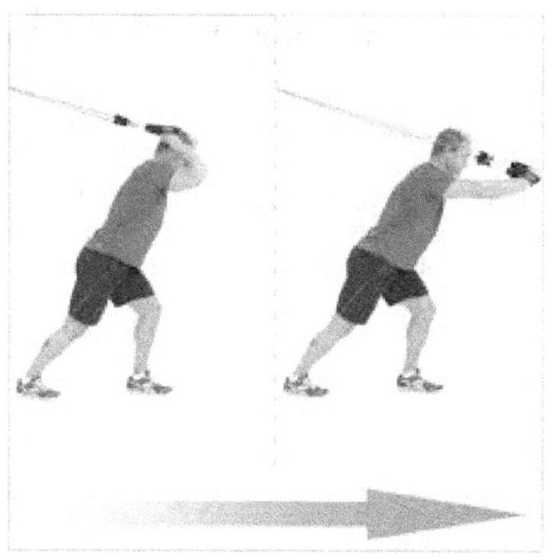

How to do them:

Step 1: Loop the resistance band through your truck's door handle.

Step 2: Stand straight facing away from the truck but with your hands holding the resistance band behind your head.

Step 3: Push the resistance band forward by extending your forearms until a point where your elbows are straight. Go back to the starting position and repeat.

Cool Down Exercises

After every workout, it is critical to do some cool-down exercises. Cool-down exercises are important because they help your body to ease back to its natural resting state. This enables you to recover for your next day's exercises without being too sore. It also decreases your chances of getting injuries.

Here is a couple of good cool-down exercises you can do:

Cat cow

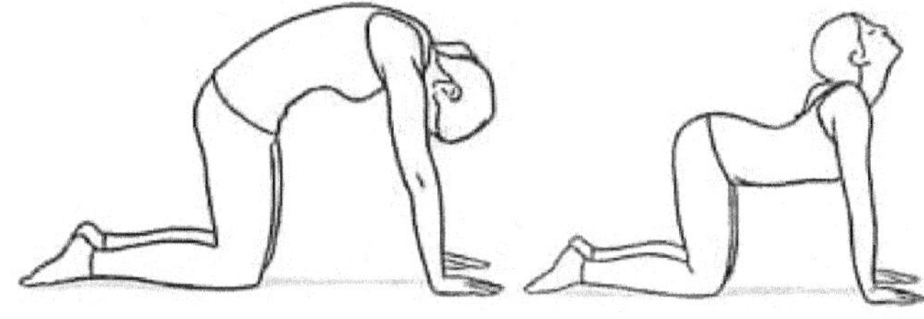

This workout is great for your back, abs, hips, neck, and spine.

Step 1: Start while on all-fours. Your knees should be beneath your hips and your hands beneath your shoulders.

Step 2: Inhale and arch your back as you look to the sky. Hold for 5-10 seconds.

Step 3: Exhale, push your hands in the ground and round your back.

Step 4: Direct your head toward the floor as you let your shoulders and blades naturally move away from each other. Hold for a few seconds. Repeat.

Standing Forward Bend

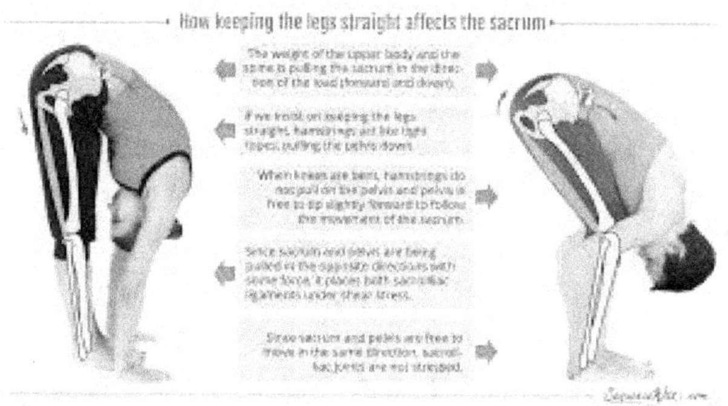

Good for calves and hamstrings

Step 1: Stand upright and inhale.

Step 2: Exhale as you bend over to reach out to your toes using your hands. You should feel it in your hamstrings. Hold for 10- 15 seconds.

Overhead Shoulder Stretch

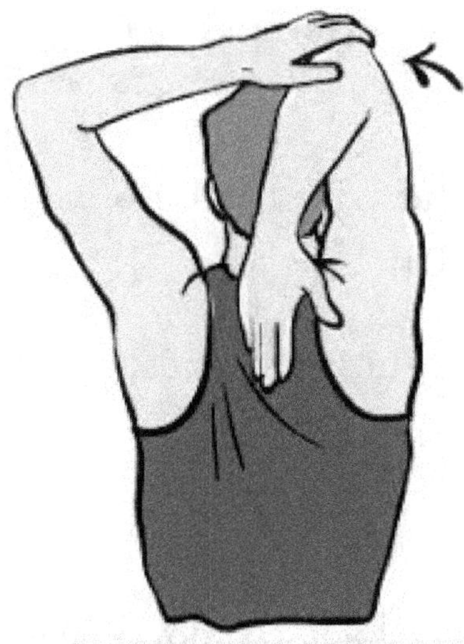

Good for your back, shoulders, and triceps.

Step 1: Stand up tall. Inhale as you reach both of your arms over your head.

Step 2: Slowly bend your right arm behind you and then grab it with your right hand.

Step 3: Exhale as you push that elbow down. Your shoulders should be relaxed. Hold for 10-15 seconds, switch sides, and repeat.

Wrist rolls

Good for your wrist muscles.

How to do them:

Step 1: Stand upright and clasp your hand together in front of you.

Step 2: In a circular motion, roll your right hand over your left, then your left hand over your right.

Step 3: Keep the movement going for 20-25 seconds, switch the direction of the motion, and then repeat.

You now have a couple of exercises that you can do while on the road. To get the most out of them, you need to create a balanced weekly workout schedule that you can follow. A workout schedule is good because it balances how much exercise each of your body parts is getting to give you a major boost in your efforts to lose weight, get fit, and be healthy.

Here is a sample weekly workout schedule you can follow.

MONDAY: Chest and back workout

TUESDAY: Core workouts

WEDNESDAY: Rest

THURSDAY: Leg and arm workouts

FRIDAY: Full body workout (perform exercises meant for different parts of your body)

SATURDAY: Do some stretches

SUNDAY: Rest

Workout Tips

Here are workout tips that will help you get the most out of your exercises:

Be Consistent

It is crucial that you remain consistent with your workouts if you want to improve your health. If on your schedule, you need to go for a jog every morning before breakfast- do so no matter how strong your body opposes. Just working out one day and expecting good results will not just cut it. You need to be consistent with your workouts to enjoy great results.

Have Realistic Goals

There is nothing that kills your morale when you exercise, like having unrealistic goals. A good example is setting a goal to lose 20 pounds in a month. You took quite a while to gain the weight; therefore, it will take time to lose it. It would also be best to start slowly instead of trying too challenging workouts or doing so much. It is crucial to do this since your body will have time to adjust to the workouts. If you do not do this and start doing too much too soon, you are likely to be demotivated because the workouts will feel too much for your body, and you may give up altogether before you see any results.

Therefore, be very patient with yourself and set realistic goals. Reasonable goals to start with are goals that help you keep going with your healthy behavior, like setting a goal to exercise every day; however, few exercises you do as long as you work out. Over time, you can start increasing the duration of your workouts.

Be flexible.

As you already know, life is unexpected. One day you can wake up at 7 a.m. to exercise for 20 minutes as planned, but there are days you will wake up late because either you are tired, or you just had a long night. If you are rigid and have to follow a structure, unexpected circumstances like waking up late will throw you off-balance, and you may find that you are not working out because you feel the circumstances are not ideal.

The thing with life is that there will always be something unexpected, and you need to be flexible enough to adjust accordingly and move on, or else you will never work out.

Be mindful of the weather as you work out.

Since you are likely to be doing your exercises outside, it is essential that you are mindful of the weather. For example, exercising in hot and humid conditions can lead to dehydration and overheating. You can slow your pace to reduce the impact of the heat or work out early in the morning or the evening when it is a bit cooler. Also, when it is cold, ensure you dress appropriately to avoid hypothermia.

Change your attitude.

Most people have the all-or-nothing attitude when it comes to working out. You do not have to spend hours working out or doing exercises you hate. Even a little exercise goes a long way in improving your health. Also, a little exercise is better than not working out at all.

Listen to your body.

Even if you have a schedule to follow, when you feel sick or fatigued, hold off on the exercises. Instead, you could opt just to stretch and not do anything to avoid causing more problems when working out when you are not feeling well.

Rest

I know you want to lose weight and get fit and so you may want to train hard or even too often. Doing this is counterproductive and will instead cause injuries such as sore muscles and joints, stress fractures, and inflamed tendons. Therefore, it is essential to rest and vary your workouts to ensure that you are not doing the same exercises that could be causing more wear and tear on certain body parts.

Be patient.

Most people who start working out expect instant results forgetting that it takes quite a while to build the kind of body you want. Therefore, do not give up when it feels like you are not getting any results. Just keep at it, keep tweaking your workouts, and in no time, you will enjoy the fruits of your hard work.

Conclusion

As mentioned in the book, the picture that most people have in their heads of a truck driver is someone who is overweight and unhealthy; however, this does not have to be you. You can change this narrative by using the guidelines in this book to lose weight, get fit and live a healthier lifestyle.

All the best as you begin your journey of healthy living!

About the Author

Nicholas Slahta is the agency owner of Red Ox Insurance Agency, a veteran owned and operated insurance agency focused on the trucking/transportation industry.

Nicholas would be happy to help you with your insurance needs and can be reached at 502-510-3030 or you can request a free, no obligation quote at www.redoxinsurance.com.

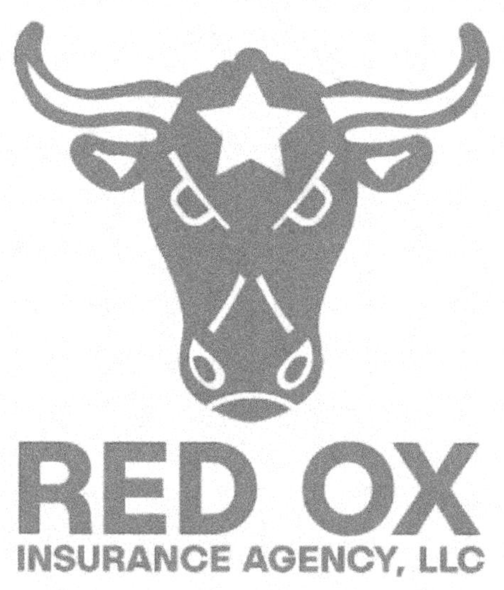

Disclaimer

Nicholas Slahta is not a doctor, dietician or fitness specialist. Everything in this book is a suggestion. Please consult with your doctor before starting a new diet or exercise program.